Intermittent Fasting

Discover Delicious And Nutritious Meals To Boost Metabolism And
Improve Health Is A Step-By-Step Guide To Preparing
Nutritious And Delicious Meals

I0135874

(Utilize Time-Restricted Feeding To Improve Your
Health)

Süleyman Guggenberger

TABLE OF CONTENT

Introduction

Nothing prevents women from achieving the happiness, vitality, and significance they desire in life. We have never lived longer than we do today. Additionally, our health practices are unparalleled. We are improving our diets, becoming more physically fit without exercising more, and figuring out how to maintain a healthy balance in our increasingly hectic lives.

There is so much to look forward to, and everything is in our favor. As we age, however, we really become more cognizant of how sedentary and youthful we once were. Simply put, we just feel alienated from ourselves. Have you ever encountered this? If so, allow me to introduce you to somebody.

Her job as a healthcare professional was challenging. It required long hours of service to the really need of her patients, as well as those of their families and coworkers, and was academically rigorous.

Due to her hectic schedule, she felt compelled to miss out on much of what was occurring in the lives of her three children in elementary school. She struggled to obtain sufficient rest. She struggled to muster the energy to leave her bed in the morning. She was gaining weight and felt unattractive and chubby. As before, she maintained her go-go-go, you can do it lifestyle. She altered her diet and nutrition to alleviate her symptoms, but she went beyond consuming too few carbohydrates and engaging in excessive physical activity. In both cases, it just got worse.

She was entering perimenopause, the five to seven years of rapidly fluctuating hormones preceding menopause. Her progesterone levels were declining, whereas her oestrogen levels were fluctuating. These hormonal changes exacerbated her weight gain and induced unnecessary food cravings. The stresses in her life only exacerbated her hormonal instability. She was resolved to alter her lifestyle because she had had enough. She stopped overworking her body, switched to a softer form of exercise, eliminated inflammatory foods from her diet, and stopped feeding it. But her weight remained stable. Not even a single pound.

She eventually agreed to begin taking a prescription medication for her hypothyroidism. She believed that by taking the medication, the excess weight would disappear on its own. not even close Her doctor, family, and friends all dismissed the weight gain and other symptoms with good intentions, saying, "Get used to it, as you are now in your forties. You are now residing in a new norm." Due to her failing health, she became discouraged, exhausted, unsure of what to do, and generally despondent.

I was that woman. My responsibilities as a wife, mother, and active doctor, combined with excessive stress, lack of sleep, and a low-carbohydrate diet, had a negative effect. I was no longer satisfied with my way of life. I requisite assistance. I eventually arrived at a definitive answer that changed everything. Intermittent fasting is the answer. I was astounded to simple discover that it repaired my body, restored the balance of my hormones, and gave me extraordinary new control over my life. To lose weight, I improved my health. So, what exactly is this phenomenon known as intermittent fasting?

In this book, you will learn everything there is to know about intermittent fasting, but in a nutshell, it is a method that emphasizes when you eat rather than what you eat. Initially, I had doubts. Intermittent fasting is such a radical and counterintuitive concept. After all, aren't we advised to consume three healthy meals and two healthy snacks per day?

The answer to this question is "not really," which is supported by a bewildering amount of clinical evidence. As my research progressed, I discovered some incredible benefits of intermittent fasting. It restores our natural cycles, stabilizes our hormones, burns fat, and regenerates our health at the cellular level. As a result, we are more susceptible to autoimmunity, cardiovascular disease, and obesity. I was overjoyed by what I had discovered. I realized I needed to make a change because I was in such poor shape and wasn't achieving the desired results.

I therefore decided to experiment with intermittent fasting. The results were nothing short of revolutionary. This weight had finally been lost. My hormone levels that were out of whack were balanced. I had enhanced vitality and laser-like mental acuity. Because I was not eating or digesting anything in the morning, I was more productive. In addition, because planning meals and snacks was no longer a priority, I was more productive overall. Since intermittent fasting transformed my life, I was confident that it would have the same effect on the hundreds of women with whom I work. All of these factors played a role in the creation of this book.

This novel book employs a strategy for intermittent fasting that is tailored to the specific really need of women. We possess anatomy and physiology that are distinct from those of men. All of this is influenced by hormones, which fluctuate daily and significantly depending on our life stage — perimenopause, menopause, and beyond. This book differs from others in that intermittent fasting does not have a single technique that is universally effective.

Chapter 1: Myths And Misconceptions Regarding Intermittent Fasting

Intermittent fasting is frequently misunderstood by dogmatic bodybuilders who refuse to change their minds and instead rely on current research to advise their clients. When a person has spent years investing time and energy in a belief, it is understandable that it actually become nearly impossible for the average person to return and question his methods.

The purpose of this article is to dispel the prevalent myths about intermittent fasting.

Like Water

The greater your investment in something, the greater your attachment to it. The process of discarding an uninteresting $50 book is more difficult than discarding a free book. Certainly, it will be much more difficult to abandon an idea that prompted you to engage in online debates, write books, produce videos, and build your reputation.

This concept is known in economics as " unrecoverable cost." This resistance to change frequently compels individuals to continue investing in obsolete ideas.

What is the significance of intermittent fasting? The majority of critics of fasting are individuals who have already spent too much money on other methods and therefore cannot see things objectively or scientifically.

"When water is added to a bottle, it actually become the bottle. You place it in a teapot; it transforms into the teapot. Now the water can either flow or crash. Be water, my friend."

- Bruce Lee

If you wish to advance, you must acknowledge that the world is changing, and that information that was pertinent yesterday may not be relevant today, or is no longer unique. Be practical and adaptable. Be water, adapt, and do not place your faith in this or that opinion. I have long held the belief that there are miraculous recipes, enchanted formulas, and superior complex techniques. Reality? Oftentimes, the best way to achieve a goal is through simplicity.

MYTH # 1 ON INTERMITTENT FASTING: EATING FREQUENTLY ACCELERATES METABOLISM

The idea that people consume six meals per day is that a high meal rate has metabolic benefits, and you should eat this way to lose more fat and be healthier. The ideas underlying this insanity have been repeated countless times. Whole books have been written on the topic of eating frequently, and obsessive people will often go to great lengths to achieve perfect adherence to this purportedly ideal frequency. With a protein shaker and six meticulously counted almonds, people meticulously prepare their lunches for the following day, which they will eat on their desk at work. Based on the thermal effect of food and a slight increase in metabolic rate when eating, the most prevalent argument is that frequent eating "accelerates" metabolism.

REALITY

Remember that the thermal effect of food is proportional to the amount of food consumed during a meal (10% of total calories, on average). Simply put, the thermal effect of consuming 2,000 calories per day is 200 calories. To illustrate, if you consume six 333-calorie meals, the thermal effect will be 33,3 calories, or 200 in total. Three meals with 666 calories? You easy burn 66 per meal, for a total of 200 calories.

MYTH # 2 ON INTERMITTENT FASTING: SKIP MEAL SLOWS METABOLISM

People fear that if they skip a meal or leave too much time between meals, their metabolic rate will immediately slow down and hinder fat loss. This misconception terrifies them more when it comes to breakfast. The expert in advertising was able to persuade them that breakfast was "essential" to start the day and speed up fat loss. " Mmmmm, a bowl of Special K snowflakes will help me lose my love wrists.

Rat research supports the notion that skipping breakfast will cause your metabolism to easy burn less energy. Negative effects were observed. However, it is crucial to remember that these small rodents have a much shorter life expectancy than humans. These animals have no fat reserves to provide energy, so a deficit must be fatal for them immediately.

REALITY

A meal or a day is a much larger part of these animals' lives than it is for us. A meal for a mouse may equal an entire day for a human. A day without food would last us approximately seven days. Even after three to four days without food, the metabolic rate does not slow.

The absence of a meal has NO IMPACT ON OUR METABOLISM (some research shows that they increase slightly during fasting).

MYTH # 3 ON INTERMITTENT FASTING: EATING FREQUENTLY PROTECTS MUSCLE MASS

"Eating frequently to prevent muscle wasting" is a nearly universal adage. People fear losing muscle if they go too long between meals, so they do everything possible to have constant access to food.

It's tiring. Sincerely, it is mentally and physically draining. Always considering the next meal.

REALITY

Unfortunately, the fear of "muscle wasting" is only warranted in EXTREME cases of differences in meal frequency, and even then, only if the protein intake is inadequate. If the dosage is sufficient, the frequency is not crucial.

If you consume enough protein, you should disregard the frequency and do whatever is convenient. The fact that your favourite fitness celebrity consumes six meals per day does not indicate that this is the only option.

In short, research indicates that the difference between three and six meals per day has no effect on fat loss or muscle retention. Individuals should select a frequency that complements their lifestyle, requirements, and preferences.

Any belief that there is a greater frequency is simply false. In fact, there are advantages for certain individuals, such as women, to eat only two or three meals per day.

THE KEYS TO THIS QUICKNESS

As in the previous example, you should consume water, unsweetened infusions, coffee, and other calorie-free, healthy beverages. It also aids in coping with a busy schedule (reading, practising some gentle exercise routine)

HOW TO BEGIN THE HALF-FAST 5/2

This variant allows 500 calories to be consumed in one or two meals during the two-day fast. For instance, steamed hake with vegetables, tortillas with lemon and onion, peppers, and baked zucchini.

Cooking vegetables slightly increases their nutritional value and "forces" you to chew.

What to select?

Eat in moderation and choose foods high in water, fibre, and protein.

WATCH OUT IF YOU FOLLOW IT TWO OR THREE DAYS IN A ROW

Extending the time between meals can be problematic and requires specialised advice.

It is the most-asked-about fast. As a result of the lengthy period of abstinence, it is typically the most expensive procedure. In addition, many experts assert that it offers no advantage over competing products.

It is believed that fasting for more than one day in a row is probably the least safe and can even increase the risk of fasting uncontrollably (such as decreased metabolism, loss of muscle mass, hypoglycemia, headaches, dizziness, heartburn, cramping, irritation, etc.)

WHAT DO YOU GET WITH FASTING?

Periodically providing the body with a "caloric rest" has scientifically demonstrated benefits: it promotes weight loss, improves metabolic health, protects cardiovascular and cerebral health, and "gives" us years.

ON THE THIRD DAY EVERYTHING SLOWS DOWN

A healthy and well-nourished person can fast for up to 24 hours without difficulty (the body uses its reserves as an alternative source of energy and thus continue to function normally). If it continues, however, the metabolism begins to slow on the third day because, in the absence of food, the body begins to conserve energy.

Instead of burning the accumulated fat, the body expends less energy when this occurs. When the normal diet is resumed, the body consequently gains weight more quickly (yo-yo effect).

HOW TO DO IT "IN THE STYLE OF SABER VIVIR"

Give your body a "caloric rest" by slightly extending your overnight fast. There is a simple and healthier way to give your digestive system a break, allowing the body time to mobilise fat and reduce fat stores.

EVENING FAST

It is as simple as advancing dinner time and (slightly) extending breakfast time.

Example: supper at 8 p.m. and breakfast between 9 and 10 a.m.

In this way, you can achieve a 12- to 14-hour fast without suffering (since you'll be sleeping for the majority of the time) while your body benefits. It is a version of the fast that I described at the outset, with a cadence of 16-8, in which you eat between two and three times during those eight hours.

STEP BY STEP

Dinner between 6 pm and 8 pm. Choose nutrient-dense foods that are also low in calories. Prepare some vegetables along with a protein source (egg, fish) and a soft dessert.

Breakfast is served between 8 and 10 a.m. It is essential that you adequately hydrate, and your breakfast should include fruit, protein, and whole grains. Take care of the remaining meals of the day.

A simple recommendation for menu design is to include dishes that are light but filling.

Prioritize water- and fiber-rich foods (vegetables and fresh fruit).

Breakfast includes coffee. Vegetables and turkey fill a half-whole sandwich. Kiwi.

3 grammes of fibre per 100 grammes of kiwi

Seasonal vegetable salad and brown rice for dinner. With eggplant, tomato, and thyme, baked chicken. Yogurt.

Vinaigrette-grilled vegetables (with potatoes) for dinner. Papillote of sea bass with onion, mushrooms, and capers. Watermelon.

Chapter 2: A "Up-Day, Down-Day" Strategy For Intermittent Fasting

Each day is either a "up" or "down" eating or fasting day according to the up/down day intermittent fasting method ("down"). You can choose from a variety of fasting and eating schedules and test out various strategies to determine which one works best for you. In up/down day systems, individuals are typically not required to observe complete fasts on their down days. On specific days, you may consume up to 500 calories. Not exactly what the original authors wrote about fasts are these programmes. Numerous benefits of fasting persist, and the up-and-down eating pattern effectively prevents the metabolic adaptation that occurs with a typical low-calorie diet (recall the

Biggest Loser study from the chapter on calories) (remember the Biggest Loser study, which you read about in the chapter about calories.) Even if 500 calories are permitted, remember what we learned in the previous chapter about insulin. If you wish to fast, create a diet that promotes fat burning, as you do not want to release insulin frequently. For more information on how to prevent insulin release during the fasting period, please refer to the chapter on what you can eat while fasting. These systems "allow" you to consume up to 500 calories on non-fasting days, but I prefer to maximise the fasting period. Therefore, if I am having a bad day, I severely fast and consume no calories (other than the negligible number of calories in a cup of black coffee) (other than the negligible calorie content from black coffee). I've discovered that restricting myself to 500 calories is more difficult for me than fasting for 36 hours. You are permitted to try out various fasting methods to determine which one works best for you; the "best" method is the one that makes it easiest for you to adhere to your fasting days. When I'm having a bad day, I drink only black coffee, water, or sparkling water from the time I wake up until I go to bed. Before going to bed, I consume nothing. The following day is an up day, so I am free to break my fast whenever I choose.

If I break my fast with breakfast, I will have fasted for approximately 36 hours. If I do not break my fast until midday, I will have fasted for nearly 42 hours.

If you are contemplating using an up/down day approach to intermittent fasting, you have a variety of options available to you. Alternate day fasting (ADF) is the most extreme form of up/down day fasting. ADF is exactly what it sounds like: on the first day, you fast and on the second, you eat whatever you want. The alternate-day cycle continues indefinitely.

The Every Other Day Diet by Dr. Kristina Varady discusses the results of an extensive study she conducted on ADF. The Alternate-Day Diet by Dr. Johnson is another book that supports the alternate-day strategy. Both Drs. Vardy and Johnson recommend counting calories on fasting days.

On days when you eat frequently, Dr. Johnson recommends monitoring your caloric intake. According to Dr. Varady's research, relatively few people overeat on special occasions, and weight loss can occur even when calories are not strictly monitored. The technique of your choosing is available for your selection. I would rather never count calories. As it is simple to count to zero, I could have chosen to observe a complete fast during my version of the down days.

On the opposite end of the up/down day spectrum is a strategy known as 5:2. The numbers 5 and 2 represent the days of the week you perform the activity. The first number represents the number of days per week that you eat normally (five), and the second number represents the number of days per week that you fast (2). On the 5:2 diet, you may choose any two days of the week to fast while eating "normally" on the other five days. On fasting days, you are permitted to consume up to 500 calories, but I always choose to consume zero. This is comparable to ADF. The 5:2 diet is advantageous for a number of reasons, as you only restrict your food intake on two days per week and otherwise consume a normal diet. According to me, one of the most significant disadvantages of the 5:2 diet is that you only restrict your food intake on two days per week, while eating normally on the other five. It is simply too much food for me to eat five days per week in a responsible manner. Even though I do not lose weight while following the 5:2 diet, it is an excellent method for weight maintenance for me. During the summer of 2015, I maintained a healthy weight by adhering to the 5:2 diet from April to August.

I suggest you try the 4:3 diet if the ADF seems excessive and the 5:2 seems inadequate. The first number, as in 5:2, indicates how many days per week you eat normally (4), and the second number, as in 5:2, indicates how many days per week you fast (3). (3). (3). (3). I find that the 4:3 diet helps me lose weight (albeit slowly), whereas the 5:2 diet only helps me maintain my weight (albeit slowly) (although slowly).

If you are utilising ADF, 4:3, or 5:2, you must consider the structure of your week. Timing was an issue I've always had with authentic ADF. Because there are seven days in a week, you fast on Monday, Wednesday, Friday, and Sunday one week and Tuesday, Thursday, and Saturday the following week. I never want to completely fast on Fridays and Saturdays, and when I do, I want to stick to a more regular schedule. Instead of using actual ADF for weight loss, I would use a 4:3 plan with the following structure: I would skip meals on Sunday, Tuesday, and Thursday, leaving Friday and Saturday open for weekend social activities. If I had a commitment on Sunday, Tuesday, or Thursday, I would either fast through it or reschedule it. (One can always choose to overcome a difficulty quickly. There is not much of a difference between eating and not eating, and I've discovered that I'm less likely to eat something just because it's available; the food must also be tasty.) When I used the 5:2 diet as a maintenance plan, I fasted every week on Monday and Thursday. I always planned a nice fast on Monday following the weekend, and I fasted on Thursday in preparation for the following weekend. This exercise regimen performed miracles for me. As with 4:3, I could easily adjust my fasting days for special occasions. Up/down day intermittent fasting plans such as ADF, 5:2, and 4:3 are extremely popular because they permit you to eat normally on certain days without having to "diet." That was also one of the things that drew me in. But as time passed, I realised I was having difficulty with both 5:2 and 4:3. I began to dread the fasting days because I had difficulty sleeping after a day without food. I did not enjoy the pleasant days as much as I had anticipated. I was concerned about my next meal, whether it was time to eat, and when I would be able to eat during the course of the day. I was exhausted because I was constantly considering food. Additionally, I experienced the afternoon slump on days when I consumed food. I won't say I'll never use the ADF, 5:2, or 4:3 approaches again, but for the time being, I've opted for the one-meal-a-day (OMAD) approach, which I will discuss in the chapter that follows this one.

As a result of the OMAD way of life, I have access to wonderful air conditioning, which makes it so simple for me to adhere to the diet. I strongly advise you to experiment with alternative window lengths and fasting methods until you find AC.

Chapter 3: Immediate Adverse Effects

Of Intermittent Fasting

You may soon observe alterations in your body and digestion.

Although these side effects are less severe, they must still be avoided.

Here are a few warning signs that may appear in the first few days or weeks of IF:

having a feeling of hunger

We are unsure if this is a legitimate term, but it is a genuine experience. This is the irritability that results from being unable to eat when your body signals that it is hungry.

As previously reported by WH, it takes practise to train your body to go 16 hours without eating, and some people's bodies may never be satisfied eating within a limited time frame.

If you consume sufficient protein later in the day or at night, you should not be hungry in the morning.

But if you are, it's a sign that you need to make dietary adjustments during your calorie-intake period to avoid becoming extremely irritable, or that fasting isn't working for you.

This is something to consider for certain individuals (such as those who exercise frequently) for whom prolonged fasting may not be desirable. Don't push it.

Tiredness or mental fog

Have you ever been yawning in the middle of the day, only to realise that you skipped breakfast?

Due to the fact that most people fast without eating breakfast, if you're consistently too tired or making careless errors due to brain fog, it's a sign that you're not consuming the right foods during non-fasting hours or that fasting isn't working for you.

Consider what you are putting into your body.

On intermittent fasting, you may eat whatever you want, but you should still eat foods that make you just feel healthy and strong. Listen to your body if you generally just feel much better after eating breakfast.

Hypoglycemia

If you experience persistent nausea, headaches, or dizziness while on the IF diet, this is a red flag that the diet may be throwing off your blood sugar balance.

As stated by WH previously, diabetics should avoid any type of fasting diet for the following reason: Hypoglycemia can be caused by IF, which is problematic for those with insulin or thyroid issues.

Any intermittent fasting plan that requires you to skip breakfast may harm your blood sugar.

An empty stomach in the morning may disrupt your entire day and prime your body for intense cravings later on.

Constipation

Are all files backed up? If you do not consume enough water, vitamins, protein, or fibre, any diet could cause stomach discomfort. Who emphasises the importance of maintaining hydration throughout the day?

People often forget to drink water during fasting hours, but remaining dehydrated for 16 hours is a recipe for (gastrointestinal) disaster.

So, if you've started an IF diet and can't get regular bowel movements (or none at all), it's time to put your plan on hold and speak with a nutritionist or doctor about what's happening (or not happening in your case!).

Chapter 4: How Is Intermittent Fasting (If) Defined?

What exactly does the term "intermittent fasting" mean? Everyone is acquainted with the concept of fasting. Numerous diverse populations fast for various reasons. As part of their religious practises, some individuals skip meals in order to devote more time to prayer. Others appear to be starving without apparent cause. In the past, people only ate when they were taking a break from working in the fields. Intermittent fasting is not one of the fasting methods described above; it is not one of them. It is neither a result of a lack of food or time nor a religious practise. Alternating between periods of eating and fasting, with each interval lasting a certain amount of time, is the best way to describe this eating pattern. The 16:8 method, for instance, recommends a 16-hour fast followed by an 8-hour supper. Keep in mind that this is not a diet, but rather a way of eating. More emphasis is placed on when you should eat than on what you should eat. Does this mean you may consume whatever you desire? Regrettably, no. As with everything else, what you get out of life is dependent on what you put into it. Clean eating is one of the three legs of the tripod for effective fat loss. Does this imply that you can only consume chicken and broccoli? Without a doubt, no Since we are all human, I believe it is essential to enjoy life, but as you well know, moderation is the key.

Unlike other diets, intermittent fasting did not emerge overnight, reach its peak, and then fade away. It has existed for some time and is still in use today (even if you are learning about it just now). It is currently one of the most popular health and fitness trends.

How to Accumulate & Easy burn Fat

Studies have shown that intermittent fasting is an effective method for shedding pounds and burning fat. But exactly how does it operate? Before understanding how IF works, the following concepts must be understood: The manner in which your body consumes and stores energy, the hormones involved in this process, and other factors.

The body either expends or stores energy. No compromise is possible.

Why is this essential? In general, if glucose (sugar) is not burned, it is stored as glycogen or fat. Does this imply that you must exercise frequently? The straightforward answer is no. Actually, 10%–15% of the equation for weight loss does not involve exercise (more on this later) (more about that later). In order to easy burn energy, your body engages in a variety of specialised processes. Your body consumes energy even when you are inactive and inert because it must perform certain functions to keep you alive. RMR and BMR both apply to this. Although glucose may be burned for energy by your cells, any excess will be stored. This storage state is acceptable. Wait! If we are either storing or burning sugar, eating less and being more active should result in weight loss. It appears to be quite easy, correct? If you are reading this, it is likely that you have unsuccessfully attempted this method. Either you initially experienced effects, but they abruptly ceased, or you lost all of them upon returning to your normal routine.

How then do I lose weight?

For a better understanding, two concepts must be grasped:

The processes involved in the storage, utilisation, and combustion of glucose (sugar) (sugar).

Where does energy get stored? How do our hormones contribute to this process?

The primary methods by which the body stores energy are glycogen and fat.

During digestion, food is broken down into a variety of macronutrients. These macronutrients enter the circulation, circulate throughout the body, and are subsequently used for a variety of functions by our cells. For example, the circulatory system transports glucose (sugar), which is produced when carbohydrates are broken down, to the cells, where it is utilised as an energy source. However, if there is an excessive amount of glucose in the blood (hyperglycemia), it will undergo glycogenesis and be converted into glycogen, which is then stored. There is a maximum amount of glycogen that the body can store. Once these reserves are depleted, excess glucose is converted into fat through a process called lipogenesis.

How does energy get used?

When our cells require more energy than the circulation can provide, glycogen is converted back into glucose through the glycogenolysis process. Our glycogen reserves are gradually depleted to restore normal blood sugar levels. When these stores are depleted, a process known as lipolysis breaks down fat for energy. Wahoo! Now that fat is being burned!

Summary

When blood sugar levels are high, excess glucose will be converted to glycogen for storage.

When glycogen reserves are depleted, glucose is converted to fat and stored in greater quantities.

When blood glucose levels fall, glycogen is converted back into glucose and reintroduced into the bloodstream.

When glycogen levels are low, fat is broken down and released for energy into the bloodstream.

Now that you understand the fundamentals of how and why the body stores and uses energy, we will examine the hormones that regulate these processes.

Chapter 5: Then Why Does A Woman's Metabolic Rate Slow Down?

The rate at which we easy burn calories (metabolic rate) slows by 2 to 3 percent per decade beginning in our twenties, according to studies. Between the ages of 40 and 60, it actually become increasingly apparent. Although the slowdown affects both men and women, women are typically the most affected because their metabolisms are naturally slower from birth.

Several natural factors associated with ageing can contribute to a woman's metabolism slowing:

More fat, less muscle: As women age, they lose muscle and body mass naturally. This also occurs with men.

Having fewer muscles decreases the metabolic rate. Sarcopenia can be caused by changes associated with ageing, such as inflammation, damage, and other hormonal shifts. The breakdown of muscle fibres occurs more rapidly than their reconstruction.

Physiological and lifestyle modifications: During childhood and adolescence, the body grows and forms bones. In addition to frequent movement, it also generates growth hormones that easy burn so many calories. As an adult, however, the body produces fewer human growth hormones, particularly when physical activity decreases; less physical activity translates to fewer calories burned.

Pregnancy: Excessive weight gain during pregnancy can have long-term effects on the metabolism. These additional pounds can cause less sleep, which stimulates the hormones that cause food cravings.

Menopause: Hormonal signals are sent to the body in order to redistribute weight to various body parts. Before menopause, excess body fat would normally be evenly distributed throughout the body. After menopause, the majority of fat deposits in the middle of the body. Changing oestrogen levels have an effect on the metabolism. Some metabolic changes may be caused by another health condition, but the majority of metabolic changes are caused by natural conditions.

Thyroid problem: The thyroid is a butterfly-shaped endocrine gland located in the front of the neck. It produces thyroid hormones, which affect bodily processes such as metabolism. Women are five to eight times more likely than men to develop a thyroid disorder, particularly after pregnancy or menopause.

Thyroid disorders come in various forms. Hypothyroidism is an example of a condition in which the body does not produce enough thyroid hormones. In hyperthyroidism, the body produces an excessive amount of thyroid hormones. Both conditions can affect the metabolic rate.

Medications: Various adverse effects can be caused by prescription medications. While some can stimulate appetite, others tend to suppress it. Changes in medications can sometimes affect the body's ability to absorb nutrients.

Although these aging-related changes cannot be prevented, they can be partially reversed by taking certain measures.

12

Second Chapter

17

Contributes to Brain Health and Function Intermittent fasting may improve memory, cognitive performance, and brain health/function by protecting neurons from degeneration and death.

Emerging evidence suggests that intermittent fasting may be beneficial for neurological disorders such as epilepsy, Alzheimer's disease, Parkinson's disease, and stroke.

Keep in mind that these potential benefits are not unique to fasting; lower inflammation, body fat loss, and improved blood sugar levels have all been linked to improved brain function.

Maintains Cell Vitality And Health

Fasting allows the body to relax and repair, allowing the body's natural processes to maintain healthy cells. Autophagy is an example of a natural process that our bodies use to maintain healthy cells and, consequently, our health!

Autophagy is the process by which our cells eliminate waste and damaged cells in order to assist the body in removing damaged cells and regenerating new, healthier cells. There is evidence that intermittent fasting increases the frequency of this process, requiring the body to exert greater effort to eliminate dysfunctional cells.

Increased autophagy may protect us from neurological disorders, cancer, inflammatory diseases, and cardiovascular diseases, among others.

Chapter 6: Human Wellness And The Modern Diet

All living processes require basic nutrients, such as proteins, lipids, and carbohydrates. They provide the carbon backbone for numerous useful compounds and produce energy through oxidative breakdown.

However, when nutrition is insufficient or excessive, the body has trouble managing the absorption and storage of nutrients quantitatively. Overeating, specifically the manner in which energy is absorbed and stored, can be detrimental to health and lead to a variety of diseases, including diabetes, cardiovascular disease, obesity, hypertension, and hyperlipidemia, particularly in older adults.

Inadequate nutrition also impairs fertility and promotes the development of several malignancies, which are detrimental to the quality of human life, survival, and reproduction. Due to the fact that nutrient absorption, energy storage, and oxidative energy supply regulation vary from person to person, numerology cannot predict the daily amounts of nutrients consumed due to overnutrition.

Modern diets include "junk food" that is low in nutrients and calories. "empty calories" refers to foods that are high in calories but low in micronutrients such as fibre, carbohydrates, proteins, vitamins, minerals, and amino acids (calories). These foods lack the essential nutrients for good health.

Due to its lack of nutritional value, this meal is considered harmful and may be referred to as junk food. Junk food is a slang term for foods that are perceived to have little to no nutritional value and contain ingredients that are harmful when consumed frequently or in excess.

These foods are considered junk food because they are high in refined sugar, white flour, trans and polyunsaturated fats, salt, and various dietary additives, such as monosodium glutamate and tartrazine, but low in protein, fibre, vitamins, and other beneficial nutrients.

These foods are low in enzyme-producing vitamins and minerals. Nonetheless, they are rich in calories. "junk food" refers to high-calorie, high-fat, high-sodium, and high-sugar foods with little nutritional value.

This concept has been incorporated into the contemporary diet of the current generation. In contrast, junk food is easy to transport, purchase, and consume. In general, food colouring and chemicals enhance the flavour, texture, and shelf life of modern diets while giving them a visually appealing appearance.

Diets are reflective of the environments in which individuals reside. Urban-industrial lifestyles have only recently emerged, with most or all people preferring to reside in towns and cities over rural areas. As nations urbanise and industrialise, these patterns change quite rapidly.

Individuals' levels of physical activity, body composition and physique, life expectancy, and patterns of disease, including cancer, are all influenced by the diverse food systems and cuisines that comprise these distinct ways of life. In contrast, city dwellers are more likely to develop chronic diseases such as type 2 diabetes, coronary heart disease, obesity, and various cancers.

Good health extends life expectancy and decreases infant mortality. Health is more than the absence of disease or physical fitness. Excellent health requires knowledge of diseases and their effects on various body functions, vaccination against infectious diseases, efficient waste disposal, control of vectors, and maintenance of clean food and water supplies.

It is essential to consume junk food in moderation, occasionally, and ideally in small quantities. It is possible to overcome unhealthy foods and processed foods.

Diet influences how the genome is expressed, regulated, modified, imprinted, and passed down through generations without altering DNA sequences. Public health is a social and political concept that aims to improve the health, longevity, and quality of life of entire populations through health promotion, disease prevention, and other forms of health intervention.

The field of public health teaches us how lifestyle choices and living conditions affect health status. It also acknowledges the need to mobilise resources and make prudent investments in policies, programmes, and services that promote healthy lifestyles and foster environments conducive to health in order to create, maintain, and protect health.

In addition to the intensity of daily activities and the storage of energy substances, nutrition, specifically the sense and absorption of energy substances, is crucial for controlling ageing and lifespan.

The causes of shorter life expectancies are increased activity and rapid development, whereas the causes of longer life expectancies are decreased activity and slower development. All community members must have a greater understanding of the health risks posed by junk food. Consuming a healthy diet requires effort. Healthy eating is commonly viewed as a component of a healthy diet and as the only means of avoiding junk food.

High-fiber, low-fat, low-saturated fat, and low-cholesterol foods, such as whole-grain products, vegetables, and fruits. Adults of advanced age can meet their daily calcium requirements by consuming calcium-rich meals with modest amounts of salt and sugar. To meet your daily iron requirements, consume iron-rich foods.

Optimizing modern nutrition and human health may be advantageous for people of all ages, but especially the elderly.

Chapter 7: The Variations Between Men's And Women's Intermittent Fasting?

The biological differences between men and women are meant to reflect the distinct dietary habits that we each choose to follow. Intermittent fasting has vastly different effects on different individuals.

Women have monthly periods and are more likely than men to be affected by hormones, especially on certain days of the month; for this reason, it is always advised to listen to your body and, particularly when your period is approaching or when you have your period, to adjust your eating pattern accordingly. Men do not experience menstruation and are less likely to be influenced by hormones.

Be sure to monitor your body's response to intermittent fasting and make any necessary dietary changes.

Examples of Several Intermittent Fasting Schedules
There are several ways to incorporate fasting into your daily routine if you are considering giving it a try.

Intermittent Fasting Each Day

The majority of the time, I use the intermittent fasting model created by Dr. Leangains, which consists of a 16-hour fasting period followed by an 8-hour eating period. Martin Berkhan of Leangains.com is credited with popularising this method of daily intermittent fasting, which is also where the term "leangains" was first used.

It makes no difference when the eight-hour eating window begins. You may start at 8:00 AM and conclude at 4:00 PM. You may also start at 14:00 and end at 20:00. Whatever is most beneficial to you, pursue it. Between 1 and 8 p.m., according to my experience, is the optimal time to consume food. This permits me to dine with both friends and family. Even though breakfast is the most important meal of the day, skipping it is not a major concern for me because I typically consume it alone.

Because daily intermittent fasting is practised on a consistent basis, forming the habit of eating according to the aforementioned schedule is relatively straightforward. Currently, you probably eat around the same time every day. It is surprisingly simple to adjust to the fact that you cannot consume food during certain times of the day. This is how intermittent fasting works on a daily basis.

Because this plan frequently requires you to skip one or more meals per day, it may be difficult to consume the same number of calories throughout the week as you would if you were not following it. This is one of the potential shortcomings of this schedule. In other words, it is challenging to train oneself to consistently consume larger portions of food. Many people who experiment with intermittent fasting find that they can achieve their weight-loss goals more quickly than expected. Depending on your goals, that could be beneficial or detrimental.

Even though I've been intermittently fasting religiously for the past year, I don't obsess over what I eat, so this is probably a good time to mention that I am not a nutritionist. I make it a priority to establish positive routines that will guide my actions the majority of the time (roughly 90%), leaving me with 10% of the time to do whatever I please. Guess what will happen if I come to your house to watch a football game at 11 p.m. and we order pizza? I am going to eat it regardless of the fact that it is outside of my feeding period.

Intermittent Fasting Once Per Week

Utilizing the technique on a weekly or monthly basis is one of the most effective ways to initiate intermittent fasting. Even if you do not use intermittent fasting to reduce your caloric intake, there are a variety of additional health benefits you can enjoy. It has been demonstrated that intermittent fasting can result in many of the benefits of fasting that have already been discussed.

The following image depicts just one potential outcome of participating in a weekly intermittent fast.

In this scenario, the final meal of the day will be lunch on Monday. You will not consume another meal until Tuesday at noon. This schedule has the advantage of allowing you to eat on all seven days of the week, while also allowing you to enjoy the benefits of a 24-hour fast. Due to the fact that you are only skipping two meals per week, it is also less likely that this will result in weight loss.

Consequently, if gaining muscle mass or maintaining your current weight is one of your goals, this product is an excellent option.

I have participated in 24-hour fasts in the past, and about a month ago I completed one myself. You have a variety of options for incorporating this fast into your schedule. For example, a long day of travel or the day after a large holiday meal can be an ideal time for a 24-hour fast. The day after a marathon workout would be another example.

Perhaps the greatest benefit of a 24-hour water-only fast is the ability to overcome the mental challenge of fasting. If you've never fasted for more than twenty-four hours before, the realisation that you won't die is a revelation upon completion of your first fast.

☐ Intermittent Fasting On Alternate Days

Alternate day On alternating days throughout the week, intermittent fasting entails abstaining from food for shorter or longer durations.

The following illustration demonstrates that you would eat dinner on Monday night and not again until Tuesday night. On the other hand, you would eat during the day on Wednesday and begin the next round of the 24-hour fasting cycle after dinner on Wednesday evening. This allows you to consistently acquire long periods of fasting while eating at least one meal each day of the week.

Chapter 8: The Lean Diet

Additionally referred to as the 16:8 method. It involves a 16-hour daily fast with an 8-hour eating window. It involves intermittent fasting for 168 days.

The 16:8 intermittent fasting method requires that you eat only once every eight hours and fast for 16 hours each day. During this fast, people typically finish their evening meal by 8 p.m., skip breakfast the next morning, and do not eat again until noon.

On the 16:8 diet, men fast for 16 hours per day, while women fast for 14 hours. If the 12-hour fast has been attempted without success, this type of intermittent fasting may be beneficial.

You might consume food between noon and 8 p.m. If you prefer to exercise in the morning, White recommends selecting a schedule with more flexibility (see the 14:10 diet).

Nevertheless, if you prefer to exercise in the late afternoon or after 5 p.m., you will still have time to refuel with a meal following your workout.

A study on mice found that limiting the feeding window to eight hours protected them from obesity, inflammation, diabetes, and liver disease, even when mice ate the same total number of calories as mice who ate whenever they pleased.

How effective is the 16:8 method for weight loss?

The (very limited) research indicates that it may be effective. The 16:8 diet was followed for 12 weeks by 23 obese men and women in a study published in the journal Nutrition and Healthy Aging.

The 16:8 diet group consumed 350 fewer calories per day, lost a small amount of weight (on average, about 3% of their body weight), and had lower blood pressure than the group that ate normally and not within a predetermined time frame.

Due to the small size of this study and the paucity of research on the 16:8 diet as a whole, it is difficult to say that adhering to the 16:8 diet is a foolproof way to lose weight.

Stress and related problems

Experts on rotundity now believe that various aspects of American society may conspire to promote weight gain. Stress may be the common denominator between these factors. For example, it is now commonplace to work long hours and take shorter or less frequent breaks. In many families, both parents are employed, making it difficult to find time to protect, prepare, and eat healthy foods together. Circular timepiece There are more reports of child rapes and random acts of violence on television. In addition to increasing stress levels, this discourages parents from allowing their children to ride their bikes to the estate to play.

Parents end up driving their children to play dates and structured conditioning, resulting in less physical activity for the children and increased stress for the parents. Whether for school, work, or family obligations, time constraints frequently cause individuals to eat on the run and sacrifice sleep, both of which can contribute to weight gain. Some researchers also believe that the act of eating hurriedly and on the run may be one of the causes of obesity.

Neurological evidence suggests that the brain's natural clock — the trend-setter that controls numerous other diurnal functions in our bodies — may also regulate hunger and malnutrition signals. These signals should maintain our weight perfectly. They should prompt us to eat when our body fat falls below a certain level or when we require additional body fat (during pregnancy, for example), and they should inform us when we are full and should stop eating. Near

Temporal cues may influence hunger and malnutrition, as suggested by connections between the brain's trend-setter and the hypothalamus' appetite control centre. Inconsistent eating habits may reduce the effectiveness of these cues in a manner that promotes obesity.

In addition, research indicates that the less sleep you get, the more likely you are to gain weight. Inadequate sleep tends to disrupt hormones that regulate hunger and appetite and may be one of the causes of obesity. Experimenters found in a 2004 study of more than levies that people who slept less than eight hours a night had higher levels of body fat than those who slept more, and those who slept the fewest hours counted the most.

Stress and lack of sleep are nearly linked to cognitive health, which can also affect diet and appetite, as anyone who has binged on cookies or potato chips when feeling stressed or sleep deprived can attest.

sad can testify. Studies have shown that some individuals eat more when suffering from depression, anxiety, or other emotional disorders. In turn, obesity and corpulence can promote emotional disorders. If you repeatedly attempt to lose weight and fail, or if you lose weight and then gain it all back, the struggle can lead to immense frustration, which can lead to or exacerbate anxiety and depression. A cycle develops that results in ever-decreasing rotundity and progressively less severe emotional difficulties.

Chapter 9: What Exactly Is Hormone?

Pistachios are recommended for replenishing adiponectin. It never ceases to amaze me how a single change in diet can have such a significant effect on hormone levels. Consuming pistachios daily improved adiponectin levels. All biomarkers improved, including waist circumference, fasting blood glucose, total cholesterol, LDL (so-called "bad cholesterol"), highly sensitive C-reactive protein, and others. What else increases adiponectin?

As a result of tampering with our hormones, we struggle with our weight each morning and have developed an obsession with the numbers on the bathroom scale. It became my inspiration. My greatest hope is that you pay more attention to your physique and are encouraged to make the healthiest food selections and lifestyle modifications.

Understanding that sustained weight loss is a result of hormonal balance has allowed many patients to finally control their weight and overcome resistance to weight loss. Weight and women are sensitive topics, and it's not just about weight loss. It is about taking charge of your life and feeling complete within. When you are energetic, powerful, and in touch with your body, you will experience favourable outcomes. Absence of bloating, moodiness, obsession, neuroticism, body guilt, and self-hatred. Finally, you can focus on your deepest hopes and dreams, the purpose of your life. You can determine what makes you just feel most alert and alive.

Chapter 10: Recipes For Healthful Smoothies

Consuming fruits and vegetables is a wonderful way to improve one's health while also enjoying one's food.

Everywhere you look, the food we consume is becoming less natural. There are an abundance of processed foods with difficult-to-pronounce additives and preservatives on supermarket shelves.

Smoothies made primarily of fresh or frozen fruits and vegetables may encourage you to consume more of these nutrient-dense foods.

The combination of these nutrients may reduce inflammation, improve digestion, and reduce your risk of chronic diseases such as cardiovascular disease, osteoporosis, obesity, and age-related cognitive decline.

Vitamins and minerals are abundant in fruits and vegetables. Fruits and vegetables, which contain vitamins A, C, and E as well as magnesium, zinc, phosphorus, and folic acid, are the best source of nutrients.

The majority of fruits and vegetables contain enough fibre to keep you feeling full and improve your digestive health, but some contain more fibre than others.

They contain few calories and fat. In general, fruits and vegetables are low in calories and fat, so you can consume more to just feel full without worrying about gaining weight.

Smoothies are a great way to incorporate vegetables and fruits for the daily vitamins and nutrients required.

Smoothies can help you shed extra pounds without requiring you to skip meals.

Smoothies are nutritious due to their fruit and berry content. Several fruits contain enzymes that assist in fat breakdown and circulatory cleansing. It may help you achieve your desired weight. It will also aid in reducing and eventually eliminating junk food cravings.

According to research, there is some scientific support for the claim that the nutrients in fruit and vegetable smoothies improve brain function and clear the mind.

Constipation is a common issue that many individuals experience. A healthy intake of fibrous foods is necessary for maintaining the equilibrium of the excretory system. Smoothies comprised of fruits and vegetables promote regular bowel movements.

In addition, they contain so many healthy ingredients that they may be an effective detox and toxin removal method. In addition, since you won't be snacking, your body won't be exposed to as many toxins. Papaya, garlic, and beets are fruits that aid in detoxification. They can facilitate blood purification and enhance the liver's ability to eliminate toxins.

Here are up to thirty smoothies designed to aid in weight loss, nourish the body, and promote general health and wellness. You can use them to break your fast, as a meal replacement, and as a delicious, healthy dessert.

Chapter 11: Quicken Weight Loss

Rapid weight reduction is one of the benefits of fasting. In one study, intermittent fasting resulted in significantly greater weight loss than a conventional low-calorie diet.

Intermittent fasting is also beneficial for fat loss and muscle maintenance. One study demonstrated that intermittent fasting increased levels of human growth hormone, which aids in fat burning and muscle building. During fasting, the body uses stored energy (fat) as fuel, as opposed to continuously obtaining energy through food consumption. This can lead to a reduction in body fat percentage.

Improving insulin sensitivity, reducing inflammation, and preserving muscle mass contribute to the enhancement of this process.

Fasting improves insulin sensitivity because the body is forced to rely on its own insulin production, as opposed to constantly consuming food and requiring more insulin.

In addition to improving overall health, reducing inflammation can aid in weight loss by reducing bloating and water retention. Inflammation within the body is associated with obesity and weight gain.

Maintaining muscle mass during weight loss can also speed up the process, as muscle occupies less space than fat and burns more calories at rest.

Overall, intermittent fasting can facilitate rapid and efficient weight loss by promoting fat burning, enhancing insulin sensitivity, reducing inflammation, and preserving muscle mass.

Chapter 12: Evidence Of If Based On Science

Even though there is substantial scientific evidence for IF's benefits, according to senior researcher Satchin Panda, it is neither a quick nor a certain remedy. Professor of circadian biology at the Salk Institute for Biological Studies in California, Panda has devoted his career to studying the complex biochemical processes of the human body. According to his study on mice and humans, intermittent fasting appears to improve human health in multiple ways, including weight loss. Before we discuss the science, let's get one thing straight: There are numerous techniques for intermittent fasting. If you search for it, you will find a multitude of options, each with its own set of supporters. The 5:2

diet consists of consuming very few calories (between 500 and 600) on two days of the week and then eating normally for the remaining five days. Another option is alternate-day fasting, which consists of eating normally one day and then nothing or 500 calories the next.

When your caloric intake is reduced, your body will utilise stored fat for energy. However, intermittent fasting differs from calorie restriction in that it may be easier for individuals to restrict calories for brief periods of time as opposed to the days, weeks, and months required by conventional diets. In addition, the form of intermittent fasting that Panda investigated may provide additional advantages. Panda has been focusing on time-restricted feeding, a form of intermittent fasting. Thus, a person consumes all of their daily calories within an 8- to 12-hour period.

Let's say you begin your day with coffee at 7 a.m. and end it with popcorn and a beverage at 11 p.m. If you practise time-restricted eating, you may eat breakfast at 8 a.m., including coffee, and finish your supper by 6 p.m. You will consume all of your meals within a 10-hour window, omitting desserts, late-night snacks, and alcoholic beverages. But this is not the end of the story. Time-restricted eating appears to be advantageous for the body in ways beyond calorie restriction. 2012 mouse research by Panda and colleagues was the first to propose this. They fed two genetically identical pairs of mice the same diet, a lab-mice adaptation of the typical American diet, which is high in fat and simple sugar but low in protein.

While both groups were provided with the same amount of food, one group had access to it for 24 hours and the other for 8 hours. Mice are nocturnal, feeding at night while sleeping during the day. When one group of mice had access to food 24 hours a day, they began eating during the day while they should have been sleeping. After 18 weeks, the mice that could eat at any time demonstrated insulin resistance and liver damage. These conditions did not exist in mice that consumed food within an 8-hour window. They also weighed 28% less than mice that had access to food 24 hours a day, despite consuming the same number of calories daily. Panda comments, "It was somewhat earth-shattering." Prior to that time, he and other academics believed that weight gain was determined by the total number of calories rather than when they were consumed. The experiment was repeated with three additional groups of mice, with identical results. Consistent results were obtained with various types of food and feeding windows of up to 15 hours, although the shorter the window, the less weight the mice gained. When time-restricted mice were allowed unrestricted access to food for two days per week, or as Panda refers to it, "taking the weekend off," they gained less weight than mice that were permitted to eat 24 hours per day.

Next, Panda's team tried a different approach: they exchanged mice that had gained weight due to unlimited feeding for mice with time-restricted eating. Despite consuming the same number of calories, these mice lost weight and maintained it for the duration of the 12-week study. They also reduced insulin resistance, which is known to be associated with fat, but the relationship is still unclear to experts. Obviously, the human body is more complex than that of a mouse, but according to Panda, these trials were the first indication of how crucial timing may be in terms of how your bodies utilise food. According to experts, circadian rhythms are responsible for the majority of human body functions. The majority of you are aware that obtaining sunlight first thing in the morning is beneficial for your mood and sleep, and that exposure to light after 9 p.m. via your mobile phones or computers may disrupt your night's sleep. "Likewise, the right food at the right time may nourish you, whereas the wrong food at the wrong time may be junk food," explains Panda. It is stored as fat rather than used as fuel, which makes sense when considering the fundamentals of human metabolism. Time-restricted eating permits the body to easy burn fat for longer durations. When you eat, your bodies use carbohydrates for energy, and if they are not used immediately, they are stored as glycogen in the liver or converted to fat. After you've stopped eating for the day, your bodies run on glucose from the carbs you've just consumed for a few hours before using glycogen or carbohydrates stored in the liver. Your body's glycogen stores persist for a number of hours until approximately eight hours. The moment you stop eating, your body begins to draw upon its fat reserves. When you reduce your eating window and extend your fasting window, you spend more time in this fat-burning phase of your metabolism. However, as soon as you eat again, even if it's just a cup of coffee with a little sugar and milk, your body reverts to the opposite mode, burning carbohydrates and storing glycogen and fat. Therefore, if you finish your evening snack at 10 p.m., your body will run out of glycogen at 6 a.m. and begin burning fat. By shifting breakfast from 6 a.m. to 9 a.m., you've given your body three more hours to use fat as fuel.

Panda discovered that his time-restricted feeding trials on humans were equally promising. In 2015, he and his colleagues attempted to implement a 16-week time-restricted eating schedule on a small sample of individuals. Surprisingly, the researchers gave these individuals no dietary advice or instructions. The participants were instead instructed to eat only within a 10- to 12-hour window. While eating, they took photographs of their food and sent them to the researchers. After 16 weeks, the patients lost a small amount of weight, an average of slightly more than 8 pounds. According to Panda, they reported better sleep, more energy in the mornings, and less hunger at night, indicating that time-restricted eating "has a systemic effect on the body." While the sample size was insufficient to draw definitive conclusions, the researchers were encouraged that the modest intervention appeared to be simple for patients to implement and maintain. It has been demonstrated that time-restricted eating reduces the risk of diabetes. After one week of restricting their meals to a nine-hour window, 15 men at risk for type-2 diabetes had a smaller increase in blood glucose levels after a test meal, indicating greater insulin sensitivity. It may also aid in cholesterol reduction. The majority of the 19 participants time-restricted their eating because they were taking medication to reduce cholesterol, blood pressure, or diabetes. After 12 weeks of eating within a 10-hour window, their total cholesterol levels decreased by approximately 11% on average. Panda then rechecked the population a year later and discovered that approximately 34% of the individuals were still willing to eat every 8 to 11 hours. "It was remarkable that they were able to self-sustain for so long," Panda continues. According to some estimates, thirteen to twelve percent of dieters regain more weight than they lost.

Time-restricted eating has several advantages over other weight loss strategies: It is simple and uncomplicated. Many individuals lack the time and resources to count calories, plan their meals, purchase specific foods, and monitor their calorie consumption. Time-restricted eating can be practised by anyone who can measure time and restrict eating and drinking to predetermined intervals.

Chapter 13.: The Importance Of Intermittent Fasting For Women Over 50 And Its Specifics

According to scientific research, intermittent fasting does more than easy burn fat. This metabolic change impacts both the brain and the body. Intermittent fasting has numerous health benefits, including a long and healthy life, a sharp mind, and a lean body. Numerous changes occur during intermittent fasting, which protects your organs from chronic diseases such as cardiovascular disease, type 2 diabetes, certain neurodegenerative disorders, numerous cancers, and inflammatory diseases. a variety of intermittent fasting diet variations have remarkable health benefits.

According to research, it may have a variety of positive effects, from weight loss and a healthier body to a reduced risk of numerous diseases and a longer lifespan. However, fasting is typically not recommended for children, individuals with severe health issues, and pregnant women. Here are some incredible benefits of intermittent fasting that science has confirmed to date:

Enhancement of Brain and Memory Capacity

Research indicates that intermittent fasting improves memory performance in both animals and adults. This diet also improves cognitive function. It aids in the fight against diseases such as Alzheimer's. According to another study, intermittent fasting also improves cognitive function, neuroplasticity, which is the brain's ability to rebuild and reorganise itself, and overall brain function.

Better Endurance Level

Intermittent fasting preserves muscle mass and facilitates weight loss. It increases endurance and enhances physical performance. Positive results have been found in these areas through research on mice. The levels of growth hormone are also elevated as a result of intermittent fasting. Which ultimately contributes to the improvement of body composition and metabolism. It also improves the long-term health of our tissues.

Obese adults can lose weight by adopting an effective intermittent fasting plan that controls diabetes by significantly reducing and regulating blood sugar levels. Recently, intermittent fasting has emerged as a novel and one of the most effective treatments for type 2 diabetes. There are numerous reports of patients who lost weight and saw their blood sugar levels improve. They were not required to take diabetes medication, and the disease appeared to be less dangerous. However, more research is required to demonstrate that intermittent fasting is safe and effective over the long term, as it requires a significant change in eating habits. Few people can maintain this in the long term.

Superior Heart Health

The benefits of intermittent fasting reduce cholesterol levels. Intermittent fasting is beneficial for blood pressure. It maintains and stabilises the heart rate. It controls the risk factors that can lead to heart-related issues and disease. When insulin levels in the blood decrease, the risk of serious cardiovascular events such as heart failure also decreases, according to studies. It is essential for patients with type 2 diabetes. These patients are 2 to 4 times more likely to develop cardiovascular disease than those without diabetes. Observational studies have demonstrated that intermittent fasting provides metabolic and cardiovascular benefits. Notable changes in metabolic parameters, such as decreased blood sugar and triglycerides, occur as a result of weight loss, and intermittent fasting can help you achieve this.

Reducing Inflammation

Researchers have discovered that intermittent fasting patterns reduce inflammatory blood markers. According to research, intermittent fasting induces the release of monocytes, inflammatory immune cells that can cause severe tissue damage. In recent years, the unhealthy eating habits of its populace have led to an increase in the body's blood circulation. During fasting, these cells enter a state of dormancy. Their effects really become less inflammatory than those of fed cells. According to researchers, fasting significantly reduces the number of monocytes, establishing a strong connection between inflammatory disease and high-calorie dietary patterns. Considering the number of diseases caused by chronic inflammation, there should be extensive research on the effects of fasting on anti-inflammation, as this affects a large number of people.

Effective for Cancer Therapy

Although little research has been conducted on the possible relationship between intermittent fasting and cancer, preliminary results are promising. The research conducted on cancer patients suggests that fasting prior to chemotherapy treatment may mitigate its side effects. It has also been supported by studies in which cancer patients fasted every other day. The practise of fasting prior to chemotherapy treatment improved cure rates. Therefore, the comprehensive analysis of cancer and fasting supports the claim that fasting reduces the risk of cancer and numerous cardiovascular diseases.

Intermittent fasting has considerable potential for both cancer prevention and treatment. As is common knowledge, intermittent fasting lowers glucose and insulin levels. It raises anti-inflammatory and ketone body levels, thereby creating a large protective environment that reduces carcinogenesis and DNA damage. Consequently, intermittent fasting not only protects against cancer but also accelerates the natural death of precancerous cells. A study conducted on ten individuals with various malignancies revealed that combining fasting with chemotherapy reduced the frequency of common chemotherapy side effects. Multiple clinical studies in the U.S. and Europe are examining the effect of fasting on the toxicity of chemotherapy and the progression of cancer.

Weight-Loss

Most people who have tried intermittent fasting have experienced weight loss benefits. It is difficult to consistently consume heavy meals, even if they are planned. Intermittent fasting is a useful option for those interested in weight loss because it provides the most amazing and simple way to reduce overall caloric intake without significantly altering lifestyle. Also, someone who consumes large portions for lunch and dinner will consume fewer calories than someone who consumes 3–4 regular meals. Intermittent fasting is a highly effective method for weight loss, as it involves the elimination of meals.

When attempting to reduce caloric intake, significant weight loss is inevitable. However, it will not benefit you. It will result in numerous health issues, including severe muscle loss. When practising intermittent fasting, the body enters a low-calorie-burning conservation mode. It is not fat that the body burns in the early stages of fasting; rather, it is water and other fluids. When you return to your eating period, the weight you lost will quickly return. The majority of people tend to regain weight lost during fasting. As a result of their slower metabolism, they may gain weight. Therefore, it is essential to practise the correct strategy and select one that promotes fat burning and more efficient weight loss.

Cleanse Your Body

Intermittent fasting may be a stressful activity, and it may take time for your body to adjust. It may initially dislike the idea, but it will ultimately provide enormous benefits. According to research, even an occasional fast has numerous benefits, and autophagy and intermittent fasting have been shown to cure cancer. It can make the treatment more effective, protect healthy cells, and reduce the treatment's side effects.

Intermittent fasting's resting period promotes autophagy, a crucial body process that detoxifies and eliminates dead and damaged cells. Giving your body a brief break from digestion and constant eating allows it to heal more effectively. It aids in the elimination of cellular debris that could accelerate the ageing process. A study discovered that time-restricted feeding, such as intermittent fasting, increases the expression of an autophagy gene and a protein called mTOR, which controls cell growth. Eleven participants were examined for four consecutive days. Another study demonstrates that food restriction is a well-recognized method for boosting autophagy, which offers numerous brain-protective benefits.

Training your body for autophagy will provide long-term benefits. Autophagy is the process of consuming one's own body. It may sound frightening, but it is one of the most effective methods for cleansing the body. Thus, the body itself actually become the cleansing facility. During this process, cells produce numerous membranes to seek out and destroy diseased or dead cells. The molecules are then disassembled and utilised to generate energy. It can also aid in cell regeneration. It is the recycling programme of your body. According to research, autophagy contributes to the immune response and inflammation. It functions as an ideal immune effector that facilitates pathogen elimination.

Autophagy is the phenomenon of cellular self-digestion that occurs during intermittent fasting periods. It regulates essential physiological processes that degrade and recycle cellular components. Autophagy provides rapid fuel for gaining energy. It provides a very solid foundation for the renewal of cellular components. Consequently, it plays a crucial role in cellular response and regulates starvation and stress during periods of fasting.

Autophagy eliminates viruses and bacteria that invade intracellular organelles. This is how it purifies the body. Autophagy is used by your cells to eliminate damaged organelles and proteins. Through this mechanism, it combats the detrimental effects of ageing.

Chapter 14: The Unpredictable Drive

While you are fasting, it may be attempting to stay alert. This is especially true if you are just starting out. With irregular fasting, there are a variety of ways to maintain inspiration and make progress. In this blog post, we will examine seven motivational methods for intermittent fasting to keep you going throughout your fast.

First, formulate objectives.
One of the most effective ways to stay motivated while fasting is to set goals. When you have specific goals as your top priority, it will be easier to adhere to your fasting routine and reap the benefits of intermittent fasting. If weight loss is your goal, track your progress to determine the efficacy of your fasting.

This will aid in keeping you alert and focused.

Tip #2: Highlight specific benefits.
Focus on the positive benefits you've observed. When you concentrate on the positive changes that intermittent fasting produces, it will be easier to stay motivated. For example, if you observe that you have more energy or just feel better mentally after intermittent fasting, you should emphasise these benefits. This will assist you in staying motivated and fasting even on challenging days.

Tip #3: Envision better well-being.
Imagining the medical benefits that irregular fasting can provide is yet another fantastic method for maintaining motivation. When you give yourself a chance to envision yourself as better, it will be simpler to adhere to

your fasting regimen and make wise decisions. This is because you will be compelled to believe in the benefits of intermittent fasting and visualise achieving your health objectives.

Tip #4: Keep a gratitude journal.
Keeping a gratitude journal is one of the most ingenious ways to maintain inspiration during fasting. In this journal, you can record everything for which you are grateful. This will assist you in remembering the positive aspects of fasting and keep you motivated to continue. You can also record some fasting motivational statements to help keep you motivated!

Read to familiarise yourself with discontinuous fasting.
To stay alert while fasting, conduct research on the topic. Acquiring a deeper understanding of intermittent

fasting will help you comprehend its benefits and how it can assist you in achieving your health goals. This information is essential for maintaining momentum and staying on track with your fasting regimen.

Sixth tip: Be swift with a companion.
Intermittent fasting with a companion is an exceptional method for maintaining a positive attitude. This is because you can support and assist one another during fasting. Additionally, fasting with a companion can make the experience more enjoyable.

#7: Reward yourself.
To conclude, be sure to reward yourself for achieving your fasting objectives. This will aid in maintaining your conviction and focus. When you reach a short-term objective, such as fasting for 24 hours, give yourself a small reward.

This could be a piece of tasteless chocolate or another book. Give yourself greater rewards for long-term fasting goals, such as a month-long fast. This could be something like a back massage or a weekend getaway.

Chapter 15: The Simple Methodology

That's it. The chapter for which you paid. This is a meticulously designed fasting method. It works so well for those over the age of 50. You should pay close attention to this.

There are various ways to practise intermittent fasting. However, they all have one thing in common: a feeding period and a fasting period.

The length of the fasting period varies among the various methods. During this time, you consume either zero-calorie beverages or nothing at all.

The feeding period varies in duration depending on the method. To prevent overfeeding, you may consume whatever you want during this period. It is recommended that you eat "normally" and not in an attempt to compensate for the time you went without food. Certain methods, such as The Warrior Diet, may require you to consume foods in a specific order.

Before discussing the SENCILLO method, it is essential to note that intermittent fasting is not appropriate for everyone. The following individuals should not try intermittent fasting:

• People under 18

People with diabetes (type 1 and type 2) without first consulting a physician

Pregnant women and nursing mothers

Individuals with eating disorders

Individuals with low body fat

Individuals with elevated cortisol levels

Before beginning any diet, physical exercise programme, or alteration to your normal habits, you should consult a physician or other qualified professional.

Keep it, safe guys!

Let us now examine the 16:8 method in detail.

SENCILLO PROTOCOL

This method consists of a 16-hour fasting period and an 8-hour feeding period. You must maintain a consistent feeding period. This means that you cannot decide to eat from 8 a.m. to 4 p.m. today and 8 p.m. to 4 a.m. tomorrow. This is done to create a schedule that is simple to follow and easy for your body to adapt to. Constantly altering your routine could leave you constantly hungry and wreak havoc on the hormones we mentioned.

This method is said to be more sustainable and easier to adhere to because you are not required to go without food for too long, and it can be easily incorporated into the daily lives of most people. For example, the average person sleeps eight hours per night. You only need to fast for eight more hours while awake, making the fast appear shorter.

For instance, if your last meal was at 10:00 p.m., you will fast until 2:00 p.m. the following day, during which time you will be asleep for a portion of the time and busy at work for the remainder; you will barely notice the time passing. Popular because you can still have dinner with family or friends before the end of your feeding window.

Critical Success Factors

1 Target Setting

I suggest that you have a clear vision of what you wish to accomplish. When the going gets tough, vague objectives such as "fit," "healthy," and "lose a few pounds" will not suffice. You must have a compelling reason for doing this, or you will likely quit. I advise my coaching clients to consider three factors.

What do you wish you could do that you cannot right now:

One month   Three months   Twelve Months

After completing this form, I instruct my clients to consider why they desire these things and what they believe will be different if they are successful. This will help you recognise your priorities.

Frequently, our goals are influenced by external factors, but they must ultimately be relevant to you.

Analyze the data and establish a:

One-Month Goal Three-Month Goal Twelve-Month Goal

2 Support

It is essential to surround yourself with positive individuals on the same path. It will really become difficult, and there will be times when you want to quit. Support from others is crucial to achieving success and could be the difference between quitting and continuing to fight!

3 Organization

Evaluate your agenda! I frequently observe individuals selecting a window for eating only to simple discover they are unable to eat during this time. Not a good beginning! Also, consider where you may have difficulty going without food. For instance, if you tend to eat out of boredom, it would be unwise to set your fasted window during the slowest part of the day. If eating dinner with your family is a regular occurrence, you should account for this in your eating window. Select your feeding window with discernment. Facilitate this process as much as possible.

Chapter 16: Can Exercise Be Performed During An Intermittent Fast?

Yes, to briefly respond. "It depends on how you feel" is the more complete response. A doctor of functional medicine who frequently recommends intermittent fasting to patients asserts that it is crucial to pay attention to one's body.

As with most things, it all comes down to developing a strategy that works well for you. The 16:8 plan, wherein all meals are consumed within an eight-hour window, followed by a 16-hour fast, and the 5:2 plan are two of the numerous IF variations.

To obtain the nutrients your body requires, you must modify your fast according to your preferred workout style and time of day.

If you just feel too weak to exercise after fasting, you should focus on your diet and exercise afterwards.

This is especially true when it comes to exercising while fasting, which has both benefits and potential drawbacks.

Exercise during a fast is safe. However, it is imperative to pay attention to your body. If you just feel too weak after a fast, you should watch your diet and avoid physical activity.

When you get out of bed for your 7 a.m. spin class, you probably haven't eaten since supper the night before.

This type of cardiovascular exercise may help you achieve your weight loss goals.

According to a study published in the Journal of Nutrition and Metabolism, exercising while fasting may increase fat oxidation1, which means that your body is using its fat reserves for energy instead of the carbohydrates from your most recent meal.

According to research published in the Obesity Journal, regular fasting intervals are more effective than total calorie restriction in promoting weight loss.

A 2014 study published in the Journal of the International Society of Sports Nutrition found no difference in body composition changes between individuals who exercised while fasting and those who ate prior to exercise. Other studies on fasting have been less conclusive.

When deciding whether fasted workouts are for you, it is best to gauge how you feel. Without hesitating, experiment with various daily exercise routines until you find one that you can adhere to.

There is evidence that exercising while fasting is more effective for weight loss than calorie restriction alone. However, the best way to determine whether exercising while fasting is beneficial is to listen to your body.

If exercising on an empty stomach makes you just feel great, more power to you. Continue doing what is effective. However, it may be time to alter your exercise routine if you begin to just feel weak or dizzy during your workout.

It is true that exercising while fasting may result in increased fat loss, but it may also result in increased muscle loss. If the body's glycogen levels, also known as energy stores, are low, the opposite of what most people desire will occur. It is essential to replenish your body with carbohydrates and protein (especially immediately after exercise) if you want your muscles to grow stronger and remain undamaged.

Avoid exercising while fasting and consult your physician about the best course of action if you begin to just feel weak during your workout.

When it comes to incorporating exercise into your intermittent fasting schedule, not all workouts are created equal. Some types of exercise are more likely than others to deplete your muscles, and as a result, you may need to eat immediately after or consume more carbohydrates earlier in the day.

HIIT and aerobics

When performed correctly, fail-safe cardio can be a very beneficial addition to your fitness regimen. And depending on the type of exercise you perform, you may or may not require food immediately afterward. The majority of the time, I advise my clients to perform HIIT cardio closer to when they would break their fast if it included strength training.

In contrast, if the cardio exercise is more steady-state, it is not necessary to perform it immediately after breaking the fast. If you intend to run slowly and steadily in the morning, you may be able to delay eating for many hours. However, if doing so causes you to just feel dizzy and weak, consider eating immediately after your workout.

In addition, it is essential to ease into any strenuous exercise while on this new diet. If a person has frequent hypoglycemia or feels ill when fasting, it may take some time to ease into a fasting regimen.

To achieve these fasting states, you must train your body. As your body adjusts to working out while fasting, she suggests gradually increasing the intensity of your workouts.

As your body adapts to steady-state cardio, progress to more challenging exercises such as:

If you want to gain muscle, it is imperative that you consume protein and complex carbohydrates either before or immediately after exercise.

If someone wants to gain muscle and strength, they should exercise either just before breaking their fast or during their eating window, as they will not be able to recover at the end of the fast.

By performing strength training during your eating window, you can ensure that your muscles have sufficient fuel to function optimally.

Do what makes you just feel the most comfortable. We must sort of strike a balance. What are your physical fitness objectives? What emotions do you wish to just feel during your exercise, and what emotions do you feel? "Something is wrong if you simple discover that exercise leaves you completely exhausted." If you want to achieve your weightlifting or HIIT training goals, it may be beneficial to consume a small amount of food beforehand.

In this situation, exercising in the afternoon or evening will be most effective.

To ensure that your muscles have sufficient fuel to perform the exercise without failing, perform strength training during your eating window.